The Ultimate Diabetic Cooking Guide

50 Unmissable Seafood & Vegetable Diabetic Recipes

Valerie Blanchard5

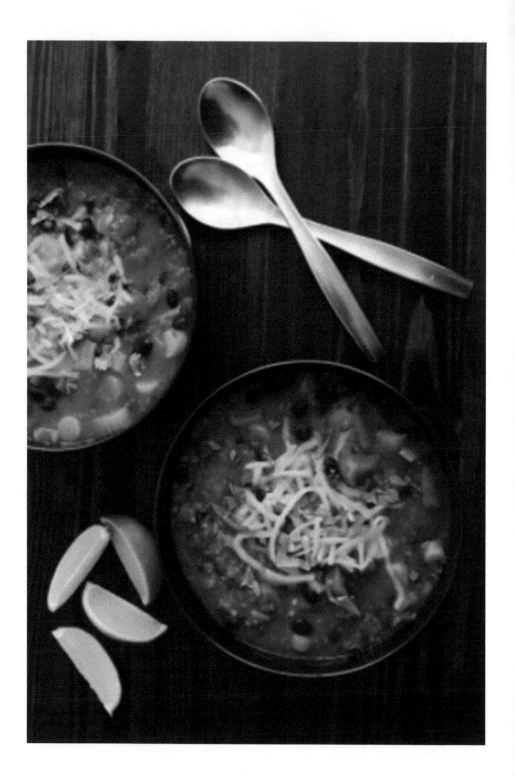

Table of Contents

Braised Shrimp

Preparation Time: 10 minutes
Cooking Time: 4 Minutes
Servings: *4*

Ingredients:

- 1-pound frozen large shrimp, peeled and deveined
- 2 shallots, chopped
- ¾ cup low-sodium chicken broth
- 2 tablespoons fresh lemon juice
- 2 tablespoons olive oil
- 1 tablespoon garlic, crushed
- Ground black pepper, as required

Directions:

1. In the Instant Pot, place oil and press "Sauté". Now add the shallots and cook for about 2 minutes.
2. Add the garlic and cook for about 1 minute.
3. Press "Cancel" and stir in the shrimp, broth, lemon juice and black pepper.

4. Close the lid and place the pressure valve to "Seal" position.

5. Press "Manual" and cook under "High Pressure" for about 1 minute.

6. Press "Cancel" and carefully allow a "Quick" release.

7. Open the lid and serve hot.

Nutrition: Calories: 209; Fats: 9g; Carbs: 4.3g; Sugar: 0.2g; Proteins: 26.6g; Sodium: 293mg

Shrimp Coconut Curry

Preparation Time: 10 minutes

Cooking Time: 20 Minutes

Servings: *2*

Ingredients:

- 0.5lb cooked shrimp
- 1 thinly sliced onion
- 1 cup coconut yogurt
- 3tbsp curry paste
- 1tbsp oil or ghee

Directions:

1. Set the Instant Pot to sauté and add the onion, oil, and curry paste.
2. When the onion is soft, add the remaining **Ingredients** and seal.
3. Cook on Stew for 20 minutes.
4. Release the pressure naturally.

Nutrition: Calories: 380; Carbs: 13; Sugar: 4; Fat: 22; Protein: 40; GL: 14

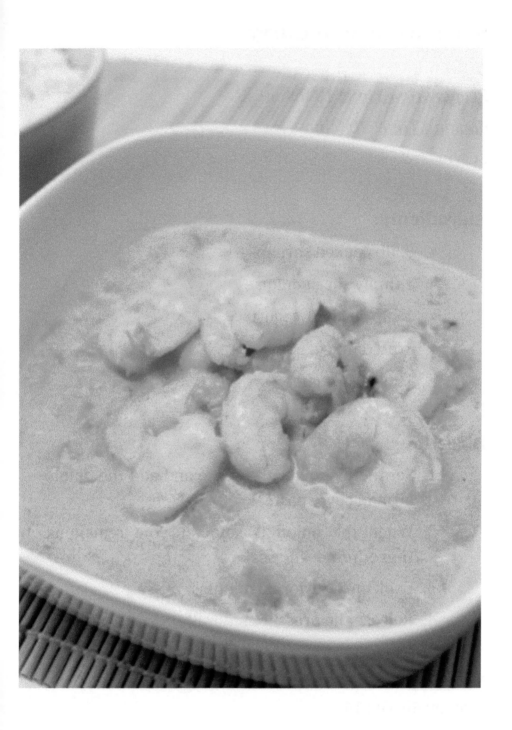

Trout Bake

Preparation Time: 10 minutes

Cooking Time: 35 Minutes

Servings: *2*

Ingredients:

- 1lb trout fillets, boneless
- 1lb chopped winter vegetables
- 1 cup low sodium fish broth
- 1tbsp mixed herbs
- sea salt as desired

Directions:

1. Mix all the **Ingredients** except the broth in a foil pouch.
2. Place the pouch in the steamer basket your Instant Pot.
3. Pour the broth into the Instant Pot.
4. Cook on Steam for 35 minutes.
5. Release the pressure naturally.

Nutrition: Calories: 310; Carbs: 14; Sugar: 2; Fat: 12; Protein: 40; GL: 5

Sardine Curry

Preparation Time: 10 minutes

Cooking Time: 35 Minutes

Servings: *2*

Ingredients:

- 5 tins of sardines in tomato
- 1lb chopped vegetables
- 1 cup low sodium fish broth
- 3tbsp curry paste

Directions:

1. Mix all the Ingredients in your Instant Pot.
2. Cook on Stew for 35 minutes.
3. Release the pressure naturally.

Nutrition: Calories: 320; Carbs: 8; Sugar: 2; Fat: 16; Protein: GL: 3

Swordfish Steak

Preparation Time: 10 minutes

Cooking Time: 35 Minutes

Servings: *2*

Ingredients:

- 1lb swordfish steak, whole
- 1lb chopped Mediterranean vegetables
- 1 cup low sodium fish broth
- 2tbsp soy sauce

Directions:

1. Mix all the **Ingredients** except the broth in a foil pouch.
2. Place the pouch in the steamer basket for your Instant Pot.
3. Pour the broth into the Instant Pot. Lower the steamer basket into the Instant Pot.
4. Cook on Steam for 35 minutes.
5. Release the pressure naturally.

Nutrition: Calories: 270; Carbs: 5; Sugar: 1; Fat: 10; Protein: 48; GL: 1

Lemon Sole

Preparation Time: 10 minutes

Cooking Time: 5 Minutes

Servings: *2*

Ingredients:

- 1lb sole fillets, boned and skinned
- 1 cup low sodium fish broth
- 2 shredded sweet onions
- juice of half a lemon
- 2tbsp dried cilantro

Directions:

1. Mix all the Ingredients in your Instant Pot.
2. Cook on Stew for 5 minutes.
3. Release the pressure naturally.

Nutrition: Calories: 230; Carbs: Sugar: 1; Fat: 6; Protein: 46; GL: 1

Tuna Sweet corn Casserole

Preparation Time: 10 minutes

Cooking Time: 35 Minutes

Servings: *2*

Ingredients:

- 3 small tins of tuna
- 0.5lb sweet corn kernels
- 1lb chopped vegetables
- 1 cup low sodium vegetable broth
- 2tbsp spicy seasoning

Directions:

1. Mix all the **Ingredients** in your Instant Pot.
2. Cook on Stew for 35 minutes.
3. Release the pressure naturally.

Nutrition: Calories: 300; Carbs: 6; Sugar: 1; Fat: 9; Protein: GL: 2

Lemon Pepper Salmon

Preparation Time: 10 minutes

Cooking Time: 10 Minutes

Servings: *4*

Ingredients:

- 3 tbsps. ghee or avocado oil
- 1 lb. skin-on salmon filet
- 1 julienned red bell pepper
- 1 julienned green zucchini
- 1 julienned carrot
- ¾ cup water
- A few sprigs of parsley, tarragon, dill, basil or a combination
- 1/2 sliced lemon
- 1/2 tsp. black pepper
- ¼ tsp. sea salt

Directions:

1. Add the water and the herbs into the bottom of the Instant Pot and put in a wire steamer rack making sure the handles extend upwards.

2. Place the salmon filet onto the wire rack, with the skin side facing down.

3. Drizzle the salmon with ghee, season with black pepper and salt, and top with the lemon slices.

4. Close and seal the Instant Pot, making sure the vent is turned to "Sealing".

5. Select the "Steam" setting and cook for 3 minutes.

6. While the salmon cooks, julienne the vegetables, and set aside.

7. Once done, quick release the pressure, and then press the "Keep Warm/Cancel" button.

8. Uncover and wearing oven mitts, carefully remove the steamer rack with the salmon.

9. Remove the herbs and discard them.

10. Add the vegetables to the pot and put the lid back on.

11. Select the "Sauté" function and cook for 1-2 minutes.

12. Serve the vegetables with salmon and add the remaining fat to the pot.

13. Pour a little of the sauce over the fish and vegetables if desired.

Nutrition: Calories 296; Carbs 8g; Fat 15 g; Protein 31 g;
Potassium (K) 1084 mg; Sodium (Na) 284 mg

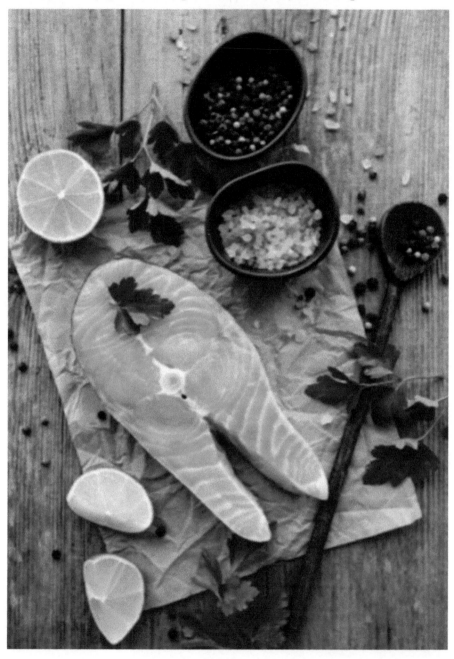

Baked Salmon with Garlic Parmesan Topping

Preparation Time: 5 minutes

Cooking Time: 20 minutes

Servings: *4*

Ingredients:

- 1 lb. wild caught salmon filets
- 2 tbsp. margarine
- What you'll need from store cupboard:
- ¼ cup reduced fat parmesan cheese, grated
- ¼ cup light mayonnaise
- 2-3 cloves garlic, diced
- 2 tbsp. parsley
- Salt and pepper

Directions:

1. Heat oven to 350 and line a baking pan with parchment paper.
2. Place salmon on pan and season with salt and pepper.

3. In a medium skillet, over medium heat, melt butter. Add garlic and cook, stirring 1 minute.

4. Reduce heat to low and add remaining **Ingredients** . Stir until everything is melted and combined.

5. Spread evenly over salmon and bake 15 minutes for thawed fish or 20 for frozen. Salmon is done when it flakes easily with a fork. Serve.

Nutrition: Calories 408; Total Carbs 4g; Protein 41g; Fat 24g; Sugar 1g; Fiber 0g

Blackened Shrimp

**Preparation Time:** 5 minutes

**Cooking Time**: 5 minutes

Servings: _4_

Ingredients:

- 1 1/2 lbs. shrimp, peel & devein
- 4 lime wedges
- 4 tbsp. cilantro, chopped
- What you'll need from store cupboard:
- 4 cloves garlic, diced
- 1 tbsp. chili powder
- 1 tbsp. paprika
- 1 tbsp. olive oil
- 2 tsp. Splenda brown sugar
- 1 tsp. cumin
- 1 tsp. oregano
- 1 tsp. garlic powder
- 1 tsp. salt
- 1/2 tsp. pepper

Directions:

1. In a small bowl combine seasonings and Splenda brown sugar.

2. Heat oil in a skillet over med-high heat. Add shrimp, in a single layer, and cook 1-2 minutes per side.

3. Add seasonings, and cook, stirring, 30 seconds. Serve garnished with cilantro and a lime wedge.

Nutrition: Calories 252; Total Carbs 7g; Net Carbs 6g; Protein 39g; Fat 7g; Sugar 2g; Fiber 1g

Cajun Catfish

Preparation Time: 5 minutes

Cooking Time: 15 minutes

Servings: _4_

Ingredients:

- 4 (8 oz.) catfish fillets
- What you'll need from store cupboard:
- 2 tbsp. olive oil
- 2 tsp. garlic salt
- 2 tsp. thyme
- 2 tsp. paprika
- 1/2 tsp. cayenne pepper
- 1/2 tsp. red hot sauce
- ¼ tsp. black pepper
- Nonstick cooking spray

Directions:

1. Heat oven to 450 degrees. Spray a 9x13-inch baking dish with cooking spray.

2. In a small bowl whisk together everything but catfish. Brush both sides of fillets, using all the spice mix.

3. Bake 10-13 minutes or until fish flakes easily with a fork. Serve.

Nutrition: Calories 366; Total Carbs 0g; Protein 35g; Fat 24g; Sugar 0g; Fiber 0g

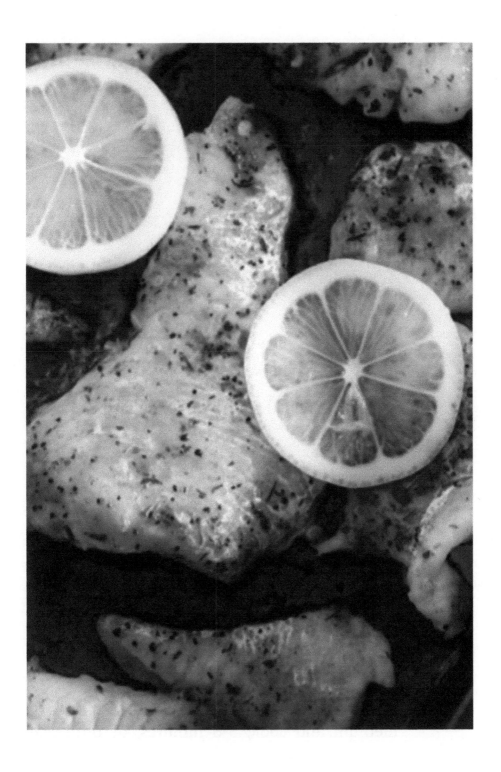

Cajun Flounder & Tomatoes

__Preparation Time:__ 10 minutes

__Cooking Time__: 15 minutes

Servings: *4*

Ingredients:

- 4 flounder fillets
- 2 1/2 cups tomatoes, diced
- ¾ cup onion, diced
- ¾ cup green bell pepper, diced
- What you'll need from store cupboard:
- 2 cloves garlic, diced fine
- 1 tbsp. Cajun seasoning
- 1 tsp. olive oil

Directions:

1. Heat oil in a large skillet over med-high heat. Add onion and garlic and cook 2 minutes, or until soft. Add tomatoes, peppers and spices, and cook 2-3 minutes until tomatoes soften.

2. Lay fish over top. Cover, reduce heat to medium and cook, 5-8 minutes, or until fish

flakes easily with a fork. Transfer fish to **Serving** plates and top with sauce.

Nutrition: Calories 194; Total Carbs 8g; Net Carbs 6g; Protein 32g; Fat 3g; Sugar 5g; Fiber 2g

Cajun Shrimp & Roasted Vegetables

Preparation Time: 5 minutes

Cooking Time: 15 minutes

Servings: 4

Ingredients:

- 1 lb. large shrimp, peeled and deveined
- 2 zucchinis, sliced
- 2 yellow squash, sliced
- 1/2 bunch asparagus, cut into thirds
- 2 red bell pepper, cut into chunks
- What you'll need from store cupboard:
- 2 tbsp. olive oil
- 2 tbsp. Cajun Seasoning
- Salt & pepper, to taste

Directions:

1. Heat oven to 400 degrees.
2. Combine shrimp and vegetables in a large bowl. Add oil and seasoning and toss to coat.

3. Spread evenly in a large baking sheet and bake 15-20 minutes, or until vegetables are tender. Serve.

Nutrition: Calories 251; Total Carbs 13g; Net Carbs 9g; Protein 30g; Fat 9g; Sugar 6g; Fiber 4g

Cilantro Lime Grilled Shrimp

Preparation Time: 5 minutes

Cooking Time: 5 minutes

Servings: 6

Ingredients:

- 1 1/2 lbs. large shrimp raw, peeled, deveined with tails on
- Juice and zest of 1 lime
- 2 tbsp. fresh cilantro chopped
- What you'll need from store cupboard:
- ¼ cup olive oil
- 2 cloves garlic, diced fine
- 1 tsp. smoked paprika
- ¼ tsp. cumin
- 1/2 teaspoon salt
- ¼ tsp. cayenne pepper

Directions:

1. Place the shrimp in a large Ziploc bag.
2. Mix remaining Ingredients in a small bowl and pour over shrimp. Let marinate 20-30 minutes.

3. Heat up the grill. Skewer the shrimp and cook 2-3 minutes, per side, just until they turn pick. Be careful not to overcook them. Serve garnished with cilantro.

Nutrition: Calories 317; Total Carbs 4g; Protein 39g; Fat 15g; Sugar 0g; Fiber 0g

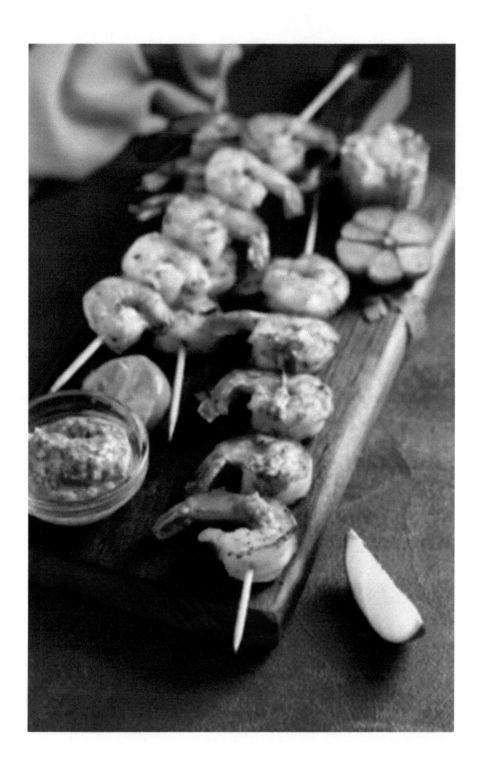

Crab Frittata

Preparation Time: 10 minutes

Cooking Time: 50 minutes

Servings: *4*

Ingredients:

- 4 eggs
- 2 cups lump crabmeat
- 1 cup half-n-half
- 1 cup green onions, diced
- What you'll need from store cupboard:
- 1 cup reduced fat parmesan cheese, grated
- 1 tsp. salt
- 1 tsp. pepper
- 1 tsp. smoked paprika
- 1 tsp. Italian seasoning
- Nonstick cooking spray

Directions:

1. Heat oven to 350 degrees. Spray an 8-inch springform pan, or pie plate with cooking spray.

2. In a large bowl, whisk together the eggs and half-n-half. Add seasonings and parmesan cheese, stir to mix.

3. Stir in the onions and crab meat. Pour into prepared pan and bake 35-40 minutes, or eggs are set and top is lightly browned.

4. Let cool 10 minutes, then slice and serve warm or at room temperature.

Nutrition: Calories 276; Total Carbs 5g; Net Carbs 4g; Protein 25g; Fat 17g; Sugar 1g; Fiber 1g

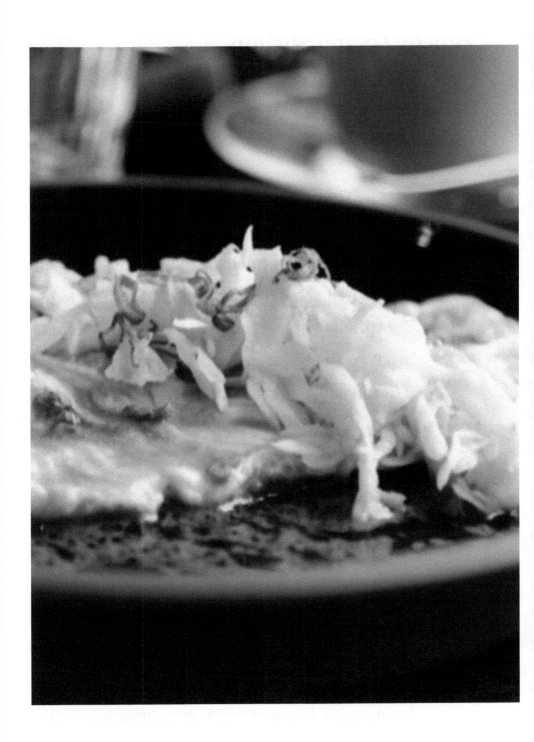

Crunchy Lemon Shrimp

Preparation Time: 5 minutes

Cooking Time: 10 minutes

Servings: *4*

Ingredients:

- 1 lb. raw shrimp, peeled and deveined
- 2 tbsp. Italian parsley, roughly chopped
- 2 tbsp. lemon juice, divided
- What you'll need from store cupboard:
- 2/3 cup panko bread crumbs
- 21/2 tbsp. olive oil, divided
- Salt and pepper, to taste

Directions:

1. Heat oven to 400 degrees.
2. Place the shrimp evenly in a baking dish and sprinkle with salt and pepper. Drizzle on 1 tablespoon lemon juice and 1 tablespoon of olive oil. Set aside.
3. In a medium bowl, combine parsley, remaining lemon juice, bread crumbs, remaining olive oil,

and ¼ tsp. each of salt and pepper. Layer the panko mixture evenly on top of the shrimp.

4. Bake 8-10 minutes or until shrimp are cooked through and the panko is golden brown.

Nutrition: Calories 283; Total Carbs 15g; Net Carbs 14g; Protein 28g; Fat 12g; Sugar 1g; Fiber 1g

Grilled Tuna Steaks

Preparation Time: 5 minutes

Cooking Time: 10 minutes

Servings: 6

Ingredients:

- 6 6 oz. tuna steaks
- 3 tbsp. fresh basil, diced
- What you'll need from store cupboard:
- 4 1/2 tsp. olive oil
- ¾ tsp. salt
- ¼ tsp. pepper
- Nonstick cooking spray

Directions:

1. Heat grill to medium heat. Spray rack with cooking spray.
2. Drizzle both sides of the tuna with oil. Sprinkle with basil, salt and pepper.
3. Place on grill and cook 5 minutes per side, tuna should be slightly pink in the center. Serve.

Nutrition: Calories 343; Total Carbs 0g; Protein 51g; Fat 14g; Sugar 0g; Fiber 0g

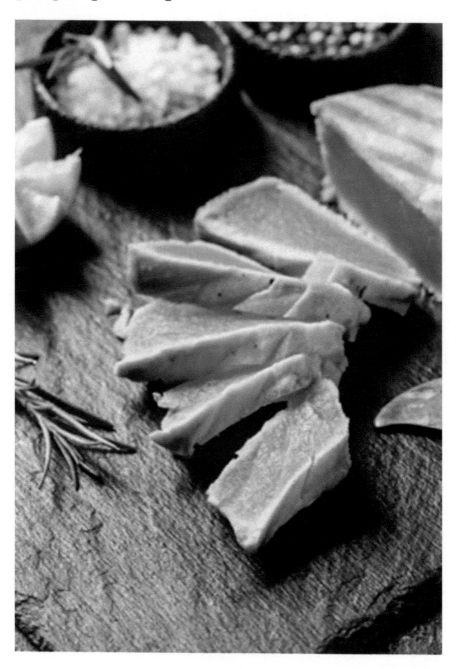

Red Clam Sauce & Pasta

Preparation Time: 10 minutes

Cooking Time*: 3 hours*

Servings: *4*

Ingredients:

- 1 onion, diced
- ¼ cup fresh parsley, diced
- What you'll need from store cupboard:
- 2 6 1/2 oz. cans clams, chopped, undrained
- 14 1/2 oz. tomatoes, diced, undrained
- 6 oz. tomato paste
- 2 cloves garlic, diced
- 1 bay leaf
- 1 tbsp. sunflower oil
- 1 tsp. Splenda
- 1 tsp. basil
- 1/2 tsp. thyme
- 1/2 Homemade Pasta, cook & drain

Directions:

1. Heat oil in a small skillet over med-high heat. Add onion and cook until tender, add garlic and cook 1 minute more. Transfer to crock pot.

2. Add remaining **Ingredients** , except pasta, cover and cook on low 3-4 hours.

3. Discard bay leaf and serve over cooked pasta.

Nutrition: Calories 223; Total Carbs 32g; Net Carbs 27g; Protein 12g; Fat 6g; Sugar 15g; Fiber 5g

Salmon Milano

Preparation Time: 10 minutes

Cooking Time: 20 minutes

Servings: *6*

Ingredients:

- 2 1/2 lb. salmon filet
- 2 tomatoes, sliced
- 1/2 cup margarine
- What you'll need from store cupboard:
- 1/2 cup basil pesto

Directions:

1. Heat the oven to 400 degrees. Line a 9x15-inch baking sheet with foil, making sure it covers the sides. Place another large piece of foil onto the baking sheet and place the salmon filet on top of it.

2. Place the pesto and margarine in blender or food processor and pulse until smooth. Spread evenly over salmon. Place tomato slices on top.

3. Wrap the foil around the salmon, tenting around the top to prevent foil from touching

the salmon as much as possible. Bake 15-25 minutes, or salmon flakes easily with a fork. Serve.

Nutrition: Calories 444; Total Carbs 2g; Protein 55g; Fat 24g; Sugar 1g; Fiber 0g

Shrimp & Artichoke Skillet

Preparation Time: 5 minutes

Cooking Time: 10 minutes

Servings: *4*

Ingredients:

- 1 1/2 cups shrimp, peel & devein
- 2 shallots, diced
- 1 tbsp. margarine
- What you'll need from store cupboard
- 2 12 oz. jars artichoke hearts, drain & rinse
- 2 cups white wine
- 2 cloves garlic, diced fine

Directions:

1. Melt margarine in a large skillet over med-high heat. Add shallot and garlic and cook until they start to brown, stirring frequently.

2. Add artichokes and cook 5 minutes. Reduce heat and add wine. Cook 3 minutes, stirring occasionally.

3. Add the shrimp and cook just until they turn pink. Serve.

Nutrition: Calories 487; Total Carbs 26g; Net Carbs 17g; Protein 64g; Fat 5g; Sugar 3g; Fiber 9g

Tuna Carbonara

Preparation Time: 5 minutes

Cooking Time: 25 minutes

Servings: *4*

Ingredients:

- 1/2 lb. tuna fillet, cut in pieces
- 2 eggs
- 4 tbsp. fresh parsley, diced
- What you'll need from store cupboard:
- 1/2 Homemade Pasta, cook & drain,
- 1/2 cup reduced fat parmesan cheese
- 2 cloves garlic, peeled
- 2 tbsp. extra virgin olive oil
- Salt & pepper, to taste

Directions:

1. In a small bowl, beat the eggs, parmesan and a dash of pepper.
2. Heat the oil in a large skillet over med-high heat. Add garlic and cook until browned. Add

the tuna and cook 2-3 minutes, or until tuna is almost cooked through. Discard the garlic.

3. Add the pasta and reduce heat. Stir in egg mixture and cook, stirring constantly, 2 minutes. If the sauce is too thick, thin with water, a little bit at a time, until it has a creamy texture.

4. Salt and pepper to taste and serve garnished with parsley.

Nutrition: Calories 409; Total Carbs 7g; Net Carbs 6g; Protein 25g; Fat 30g; Sugar 3g; Fiber 1g

Mediterranean Fish Fillets

Preparation Time: 10 minutes

Cooking Time: 3 minutes

Servings: _4_

Ingredients:

- 4 cod fillets
- 1 lb. grape tomatoes, halved
- 1 cup olives, pitted and sliced
- 2 tbsp. capers
- 1 tsp. dried thyme
- 2 tbsp. olive oil
- 1 tsp. garlic, minced
- Pepper
- Salt

Directions:

1. Pour 1 cup water into the instant pot then place steamer rack in the pot.
2. Spray heat-safe baking dish with cooking spray.
3. Add half grape tomatoes into the dish and season with pepper and salt.

4. Arrange fish fillets on top of cherry tomatoes. Drizzle with oil and season with garlic, thyme, capers, pepper, and salt.

5. Spread olives and remaining grape tomatoes on top of fish fillets.

6. Place dish on top of steamer rack in the pot.

7. Seal pot with a lid and select manual and cook on high for 3 minutes.

8. Once done, release pressure using quick release. Remove lid.

9. Serve and enjoy.

Nutrition: Calories 212; Fat 11.9 g; Carbohydrates 7.1 g; Sugar 3 g; Protein 21.4 g; Cholesterol 55 mg

Brussels Sprouts

Preparation Time: 5 minutes

Cooking Time: 3 minutes

Servings: *5*

Ingredients:

- 1 tsp. extra-virgin olive oil
- 1 lb. halved Brussels sprouts
- 3 tbsps. apple cider vinegar
- 3 tbsps. gluten-free tamari soy sauce
- 3 tbsps. chopped sun-dried tomatoes

Directions:

1. Select the "Sauté" function on your Instant Pot, add oil and allow the pot to get hot.
2. Cancel the "Sauté" function and add the Brussels sprouts.
3. Stir well and allow the sprouts to cook in the residual heat for 2-3 minutes.
4. Add the tamari soy sauce and vinegar, and then stir.
5. Cover the Instant Pot, sealing the pressure valve by pointing it to "Sealing."

6. Select the "Manual, High Pressure" setting and cook for 3 minutes.

7. Once the cook cycle is done, do a quick pressure release, and then stir in the chopped sun-dried tomatoes.

8. Serve immediately.

Nutrition: 62 Calories; 10g Carbohydrates; 1g Fat

Garlic and Herb Carrots

Preparation Time: 2 minutes

Cooking Time: 18 minutes

Servings: *3*

Ingredients:

- 2 tbsps. butter
- 1 lb. baby carrots
- 1 cup water
- 1 tsp. fresh thyme or oregano
- 1 tsp. minced garlic
- Black pepper
- Coarse sea salt

Directions:

1. Fill water to the inner pot of the Instant Pot, and then put in a steamer basket.
2. Layer the carrots into the steamer basket.
3. Close and seal the lid, with the pressure vent in the "Sealing" position.
4. Select the "Steam" setting and cook for 2 minutes on high pressure.

5. Quick release the pressure and then carefully remove the steamer basket with the steamed carrots, discarding the water.

6. Add butter to the inner pot of the Instant Pot and allow it to melt on the "Sauté" function.

7. Add garlic and sauté for 30 seconds, and then add the carrots. Mix well.

8. Stir in the fresh herbs, and cook for 2-3 minutes.

9. Season with salt and black pepper, and the transfer to a **Serving** bowl.

10.   Serve warm and enjoy!

Nutrition: 122 Calories; 12g Carbohydrates; 7g Fat

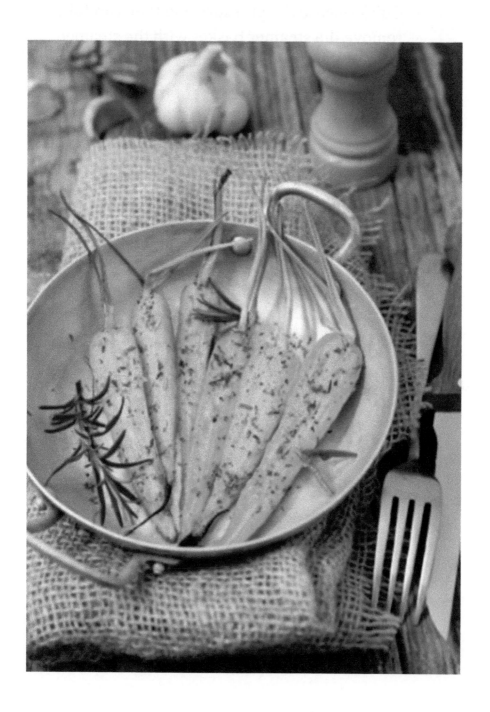

Cilantro Lime Drumsticks

Preparation Time: 5 minutes

Cooking Time: 15 minutes

Servings: 6

Ingredients:

- 1 tbsp. olive oil
- 6 chicken drumsticks
- 4 minced garlic cloves
- ½ cup low-sodium chicken broth
- 1 tsp. cayenne pepper
- 1 tsp. crushed red peppers
- 1 tsp. fine sea salt
- Juice of 1 lime

To Serve:

- 2 tbsp. chopped cilantro
- Extra lime zest

Directions:

1. Pour olive oil to the Instant Pot and set it on the "Sauté" function.

2. Once the oil is hot adding the chicken drumsticks, and season them well.

3. Using tongs, stir the drumsticks and brown the drumsticks for 2 minutes per side.

4. Add the lime juice, fresh cilantro, and chicken broth to the pot.

5. Lock and seal the lid, turning the pressure valve to "Sealing."

6. Cook the drumsticks on the "Manual, High Pressure" setting for 9 minutes.

7. Once done let the pressure release naturally.

8. Carefully transfer the drumsticks to an aluminum-foiled baking sheet and broil them in the oven for 3-5 minutes until golden brown.

9. Serve warm, garnished with more cilantro and lime zest.

Nutrition: 480 Calories; 3.3g Carbohydrates; 29g Fat

Eggplant Spread

Preparation Time: 5 minutes

Cooking Time: 18 minutes

Servings: *5*

Ingredients:

- 4 tbsps. extra-virgin olive oil
- 2 lbs. eggplant
- 4 skin-on garlic cloves
- ½ cup water
- ¼ cup pitted black olives
- 3 sprigs fresh thyme
- Juice of 1 lemon
- 1 tbsp. tahini
- 1 tsp. sea salt
- Fresh extra-virgin olive oil

Directions:

1. Peel the eggplant in alternating stripes, leaving some areas with skin and some with no skin.
2. Slice into big chunks and layer at the bottom of your Instant Pot.

3. Add olive oil to the pot, and on the "Sauté" function, fry and caramelize the eggplant on one side, about 5 minutes.

4. Add in the garlic cloves with the skin on.

5. Flip over the eggplant and then add in the remaining uncooked eggplant chunks, salt, and water.

6. Close the lid, ensure the pressure release valve is set to "Sealing."

7. Cook for 5 minutes on the "Manual, High Pressure" setting.

8. Once done, carefully open the pot by quick releasing the pressure through the steam valve.

9. Discard most of the brown cooking liquid.

10. Remove the garlic cloves and peel them.

11. Add the lemon juice, tahini, cooked and fresh garlic cloves and pitted black olives to the pot.

12. Using a hand-held immersion blender, process all the Ingredients until smooth.

13. Pour out the spread into a Serving dish and season with fresh thyme, whole black olives and some extra-virgin olive oil, prior to serving.

Nutrition: 155 Calories; 16.8g Carbohydrates; 11.7g Fat

Carrot Hummus

Preparation Time: 15 minutes

Cooking Time: 10 minutes

Servings: 2

Ingredients:

- 1 chopped carrot
- 2 oz. cooked chickpeas
- 1 tsp. lemon juice
- 1 tsp. tahini
- 1 tsp. fresh parsley

Directions:

1. Place the carrot and chickpeas in your Instant Pot.
2. Add a cup of water, seal, cook for 10 minutes on Stew.
3. Depressurize naturally. Blend with the remaining Ingredients.

Nutrition: 58 Calories; 8g Carbohydrates; 2g Fat

Vegetable Rice Pilaf

Preparation Time: *5 minutes*

Cooking Time: 25 minutes

Servings: 6

Ingredients:

- 1 tablespoon olive oil
- ½ medium yellow onion, diced
- 1 cup uncooked long-grain brown rice
- 2 cloves minced garlic
- ½ teaspoon dried basil
- Salt and pepper
- 2 cups fat-free chicken broth
- 1 cup frozen mixed veggies

Directions:

1. Cook oil in a large skillet over medium heat.
2. Add the onion and sauté for 3 minutes until translucent.
3. Stir in the rice and cook until lightly toasted.
4. Add the garlic, basil, salt, and pepper then stir to combined.

5. Stir in the chicken broth then bring to a boil.

6. Decrease heat and simmer, covered, for 10 minutes.

7. Stir in the frozen veggies then cover and cook for another 10 minutes until heated through. Serve hot.

Nutrition: 90 Calories; 12.6g Carbohydrates; 2.2g Fiber

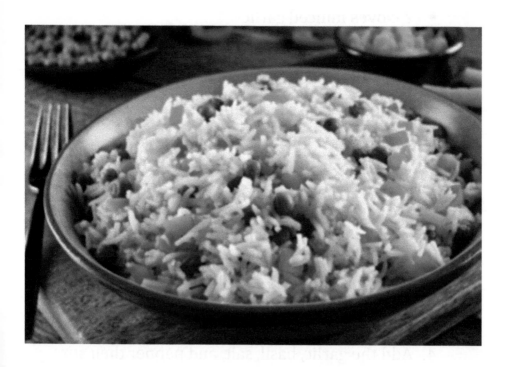

Curry Roasted Cauliflower Florets

Preparation Time: 5 minutes

Cooking Time: 25 minutes

Servings: 6

Ingredients:

- 8 cups cauliflower florets
- 2 tablespoons olive oil
- 1 teaspoon curry powder
- ½ teaspoon garlic powder
- Salt and pepper

Directions:

1. Prep the oven to 425°F and line a baking sheet with foil.
2. Toss the cauliflower with the olive oil and spread on the baking sheet.
3. Sprinkle with curry powder, garlic powder, salt, and pepper.
4. Roast for 25 minutes or until just tender. Serve hot.

Nutrition: 75 Calories; 7.4g Carbohydrates; 3.5g Fiber

Mushroom Barley Risotto

Preparation Time: 5 minutes

Cooking Time: 25 minutes

Servings: *8*

Ingredients:

- 4 cups fat-free beef broth
- 2 tablespoons olive oil
- 1 small onion, diced well
- 2 cloves minced garlic
- 8 ounces thinly sliced mushrooms
- ¼ tsp dried thyme
- Salt and pepper
- 1 cup pearled barley
- ½ cup dry white wine

Directions:

1. Heat the beef broth in a medium saucepan and keep it warm.
2. Heat the oil in a large, deep skillet over medium heat.
3. Add the onions and garlic and sauté for 2 minutes then stir in the mushrooms and thyme.

4. Season with salt and pepper and sauté for 2 minutes more.

5. Add the barley and sauté for 1 minute then pour in the wine.

6. Ladle about ½ cup of beef broth into the skillet and stir well to combine.

7. Cook until most of the broth has been absorbed then add another ladle.

8. Repeat until you have used all of the broth and the barley is cooked to al dente.

9. Season and serve hot.

Nutrition: 155 Calories; 21.9g Carbohydrates; 4.4g Fiber

Braised Summer Squash

Preparation Time: 10 minutes

Cooking Time: 20 minutes

Servings: 6

Ingredients:

- 3 tablespoons olive oil
- 3 cloves minced garlic
- ¼ teaspoon crushed red pepper flakes
- 1-pound summer squash, sliced
- 1-pound zucchini, sliced
- 1 teaspoon dried oregano
- Salt and pepper

Directions:

1. Cook oil in a large skillet over medium heat.
2. Add the garlic and crushed red pepper and cook for 2 minutes.
3. Add the summer squash and zucchini and cook for 15 minutes, stirring often, until just tender.
4. Stir in the oregano then season with salt and pepper to taste. serve hot.

Nutrition: 90 Calories; 6.2g Carbohydrates; 1.8g Fiber

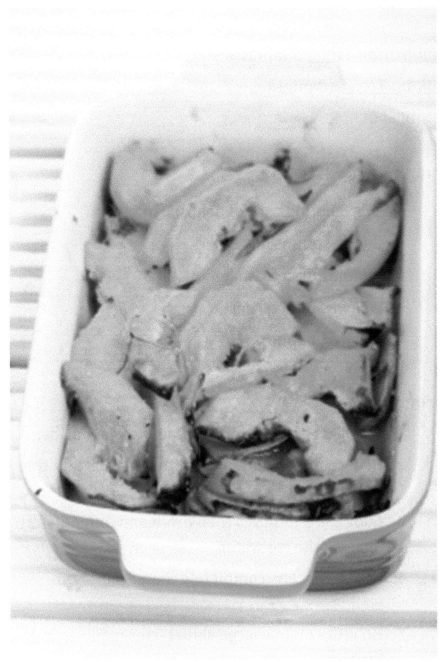

Lemon Garlic Green Beans

Preparation Time: 5 minutes

Cooking Time: 10 minutes

Servings: *6*

Ingredients:

- 1 1/2 pounds green beans, trimmed
- 2 tablespoons olive oil
- 1 tablespoon fresh lemon juice
- 2 cloves minced garlic
- Salt and pepper

Directions:

1. Fill a large bowl with ice water and set aside.
2. Bring a pot of salted water to boil then add the green beans.
3. Cook for 3 minutes then drain and immediately place in the ice water.
4. Cool the beans completely then drain them well.
5. Heat the oil in a large skillet over medium-high heat.

6. Add the green beans, tossing to coat, then add the lemon juice, garlic, salt, and pepper.

7. Sauté for 3 minutes until the beans are tender-crisp then serve hot.

Nutrition: Calories 75; Total Fat 4.8g; Saturated Fat 0.7g; Total Carbs 8.5g; Net Carbs 4.6g; Protein 2.1g; Sugar 1.7g; Fiber 3.9g; Sodium 7mg

Brown Rice & Lentil Salad

Preparation Time: 10 minutes

Cooking Time: 10 minutes

Servings: *4*

Ingredients:

- 1 cup water
- 1/2 cup instant brown rice
- 2 tablespoons olive oil
- 2 tablespoons red wine vinegar
- 1 tablespoon Dijon mustard
- 1 tablespoon minced onion
- 1/2 teaspoon paprika
- Salt and pepper
- 1 (15-ounce) can brown lentils, rinsed and drained
- 1 medium carrot, shredded
- 2 tablespoons fresh chopped parsley

Directions:

1. Stir together the water and instant brown rice in a medium saucepan.

2. Bring to a boil then simmer for 10 minutes, covered.

3. Remove from heat and set aside while you prepare the salad.

4. Whisk together the olive oil, vinegar, Dijon mustard, onion, paprika, salt, and pepper in a medium bowl.

5. Toss in the cooked rice, lentils, carrots, and parsley.

6. Adjust seasoning to taste then stir well and serve warm.

Nutrition: Calories 145; Total Fat 7.7g; Saturated Fat 1g; Total Carbs 13.1g; Net Carbs 10.9g; Protein 6g; Sugar 1g; Fiber 2.2g; Sodium 57mg

Mashed Butternut Squash

Preparation Time: 5 minutes

Cooking Time: 25 minutes

Servings: 6

Ingredients:

- 3 pounds whole butternut squash (about 2 medium)
- 2 tablespoons olive oil
- Salt and pepper

Directions:

1. Preheat the oven to 400F and line a baking sheet with parchment.
2. Cut the squash in half and remove the seeds.
3. Cut the squash into cubes and toss with oil then spread on the baking sheet.
4. Roast for 25 minutes until tender then place in a food processor.
5. Blend smooth then season with salt and pepper to taste.

Nutrition: Calories 90; Total Fat 4.8g; Saturated Fat 0.7g; Total Carbs 12.3g; Net Carbs 10.2g; Protein 1.1g; Sugar 2.3g; Fiber 2.1g; Sodium 4mg

Cilantro Lime Quinoa

Preparation Time: 5 minutes

Cooking Time: 25 minutes

Servings: 6

Ingredients:

- 1 cup uncooked quinoa
- 1 tablespoon olive oil
- 1 medium yellow onion, diced
- 2 cloves minced garlic
- 1 (4-ounce) can diced green chiles, drained
- 1 1/2 cups fat-free chicken broth
- ¾ cup fresh chopped cilantro
- 1/2 cup sliced green onion
- 2 tablespoons lime juice
- Salt and pepper

Directions:

1. Rinse the quinoa thoroughly in cool water using a fine mesh sieve.
2. Heat the oil in a large saucepan over medium heat.

3. Add the onion and sauté for 2 minutes then stir in the chile and garlic.

4. Cook for 1 minute then stir in the quinoa and chicken broth.

5. Bring to a boil then reduce heat and simmer, covered, until the quinoa absorbs the liquid – about 20 to 25 minutes.

6. Remove from heat then stir in the cilantro, green onions, and lime juice.

7. Season with salt and pepper to taste and serve hot.

Nutrition: Calories 150; Total Fat 4.1g; Saturated Fat 0.5g; Total Carbs 22.5g; Net Carbs 19.8g; Protein 6g; Sugar 1.7g; Fiber 2.7g; Sodium 179mg

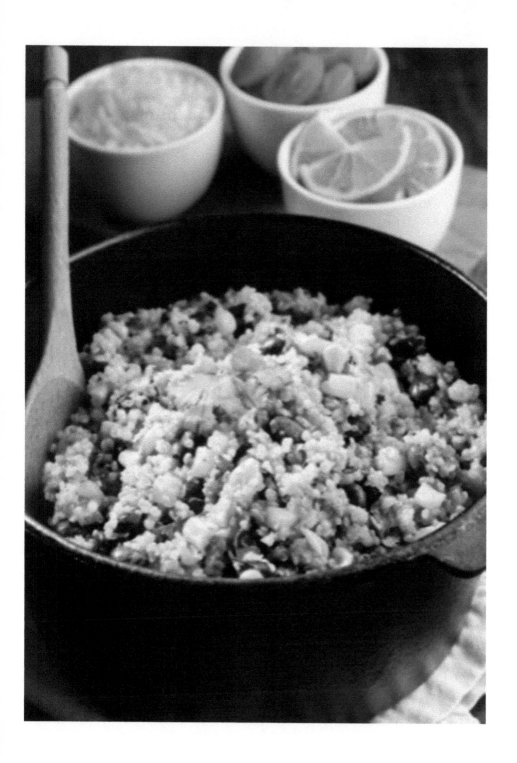

Oven-Roasted Veggies

Preparation Time: 5 minutes

Cooking Time: 25 minutes

Servings: 6

Ingredients:

- 1 pound cauliflower florets
- 1/2-pound broccoli florets
- 1 large yellow onion, cut into chunks
- 1 large red pepper, cored and chopped
- 2 medium carrots, peeled and sliced
- 2 tablespoons olive oil
- 2 tablespoons apple cider vinegar
- Salt and pepper

Directions:

1. Preheat the oven to 425F and line a large rimmed baking sheet with parchment.
2. Spread the veggies on the baking sheet and drizzle with oil and vinegar.
3. Toss well and season with salt and pepper.

4. Spread the veggies in a single layer then roast for 20 to 25 minutes, stirring every 10 minutes, until tender.

5. Adjust seasoning to taste and serve hot.

Nutrition: Calories 100; Total Fat 5g; Saturated Fat 0.7g; Total Carbs 12.4g; Net Carbs 8.2g; Protein 3.2g; Sugar 5.5g; Fiber 4.2g; Sodium 51mg

Parsley Tabbouleh

Preparation Time: 5 minutes

Cooking Time: 25 minutes

Servings: 6

Ingredients:

- 1 cup water
- 1/2 cup bulgur
- ¼ cup fresh lemon juice
- 2 tablespoons olive oil
- 2 cloves minced garlic
- Salt and pepper
- 2 cups fresh chopped parsley
- 2 medium tomatoes, died
- 1 small cucumber, diced
- ¼ cup fresh chopped mint

Directions:

1. Bring the water and bulgur to a boil in a small saucepan then remove from heat.
2. Cover and let stand until the water are fully absorbed, about 25 minutes.

3. Meanwhile, whisk together the lemon juice, olive oil, garlic, salt, and pepper in a medium bowl.

4. Toss in the cooked bulgur along with the parsley, tomatoes, cucumber, and mint.

5. Season with salt and pepper to taste and serve.

Nutrition: Calories 110; Total Fat 5.3g; Saturated Fat 0.9g; Total Carbs 14.4g; Net Carbs 10.5g; Protein 3g; Sugar 2.4g; Fiber 3.9g; Sodium 21mg

Garlic Sautéed Spinach

Preparation Time: 5 minutes

Cooking Time: 10 minutes

Servings: _4_

Ingredients:

- 1 1/2 tablespoons olive oil
- 4 cloves minced garlic
- 6 cups fresh baby spinach
- Salt and pepper

Directions:

1. Heat the oil in a large skillet over medium-high heat.
2. Add the garlic and cook for 1 minute.
3. Stir in the spinach and season with salt and pepper.
4. Sauté for 1 to 2 minutes until just wilted. Serve hot.

Nutrition: Calories 60; Total Fat 5.5g; Saturated Fat 0.8g; Total Carbs 2.6g; Net Carbs 1.5g; Protein 1.5g; Sugar 0.2g; Fiber 1.1g; Sodium 36mg

French Lentils

Preparation Time: 5 minutes

Cooking Time: 25 minutes

Servings: *10*

Ingredients:

- 2 tablespoons olive oil
- 1 medium onion, diced
- 1 medium carrot, peeled and diced
- 2 cloves minced garlic
- 5 1/2 cups water
- 2 ¼ cups French lentils, rinsed and drained
- 1 teaspoon dried thyme
- 2 small bay leaves
- Salt and pepper

Directions:

1. Heat the oil in a large saucepan over medium heat.
2. Add the onions, carrot, and garlic and sauté for 3 minutes.

3. Stir in the water, lentils, thyme, and bay leaves – season with salt.

4. Bring to a boil then reduce to a simmer and cook until tender, about 20 minutes.

5. Drain any excess water and adjust seasoning to taste. Serve hot.

Nutrition: Calories 185; Total Fat 3.3g; Saturated Fat 0.5g; Total Carbs 27.9; Net Carbs 14.2g; Protein 11.4g; Sugar 1.7g; Fiber 13.7g; Sodium 11mg

Grain-Free Berry Cobbler

Preparation Time: 5 minutes

Cooking Time: 25 minutes

Servings: *10*

Ingredients:

- 4 cups fresh mixed berries
- 1/2 cup ground flaxseed
- ¼ cup almond meal
- ¼ cup unsweetened shredded coconut
- 1/2 tablespoon baking powder
- 1 teaspoon ground cinnamon
- ¼ teaspoon salt
- Powdered stevia, to taste
- 6 tablespoons coconut oil

Directions:

1. Preheat the oven to 375F and lightly grease a 10-inch cast-iron skillet.
2. Spread the berries on the bottom of the skillet.
3. Whisk together the dry **Ingredients** in a mixing bowl.

4. Cut in the coconut oil using a fork to create a crumbled mixture.

5. Spread the crumble over the berries and bake for 25 minutes until hot and bubbling.

6. Cool the cobbler for 5 to 10 minutes before serving.

Nutrition: Calories 215; Total Fat 16.8g; Saturated Fat 10.4g; Total Carbs 13.1g; Net Carbs 6.7g; Protein 3.7g; Sugar 5.3g; Fiber 6.4g; Sodium 61mg

Coffee-Steamed Carrots

Preparation Time: 10 minutes

Cooking Time: 3 minutes

Servings: *4*

Ingredients:

- 1 cup brewed coffee
- 1 teaspoon light brown sugar
- ½ teaspoon kosher salt
- Freshly ground black pepper
- 1-pound baby carrots
- Chopped fresh parsley
- 1 teaspoon grated lemon zest

Directions:

1. Pour the coffee into the electric pressure cooker. Stir in the brown sugar, salt, and pepper. Add the carrots.
2. Close the pressure cooker. Set to sealing.
3. Cook on high pressure for minutes.
4. Once complete, click Cancel and quick release the pressure.
5. Once the pin drops, open and remove the lid.

6. Using a slotted spoon, portion carrots to a **Serving** bowl. Topped with the parsley and lemon zest, and serve.

**Nutrition:** 51 Calories; 12g Carbohydrates; 4g Fiber

Rosemary Potatoes

Preparation Time: 5 minutes

Cooking Time: 25 minutes

Servings: *2*

Ingredients:

- 1lb red potatoes
- 1 cup vegetable stock
- 2tbsp olive oil
- 2tbsp rosemary sprigs

Directions:

1. Situate potatoes in the steamer basket and add the stock into the Instant Pot.
2. Steam the potatoes in your Instant Pot for 15 minutes.
3. Depressurize and pour away the remaining stock.
4. Set to sauté and add the oil, rosemary, and potatoes.
5. Cook until brown.

Nutrition: Per serving: 195 Calories; 31g Carbohydrates; 1g Fat

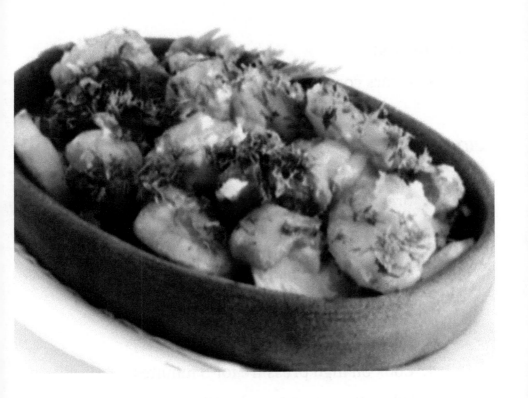

Corn on the Cob

Preparation Time: 10 minutes

Cooking Time: 5 minutes

Servings: *12*

Ingredients:

- 6 ears corn

Directions:

1. Take off husks and silk from the corn. Cut or break each ear in half.

2. Pour 1 cup of water into the bottom of the electric pressure cooker. Insert a wire rack or trivet.

3. Place the corn upright on the rack, cut-side down. Seal lid of the pressure cooker.

4. Cook on high pressure for 5 minutes.

5. When its complete, select Cancel and quick release the pressure.

6. When pin drops, unlock and take off lid.

7. Pull out the corn from the pot. Season as desired and serve immediately.

Nutrition: 62 Calories; 14g Carbohydrates; 1g Fiber

Chili Lime Salmon

Preparation Time: 6 minutes

Cooking Time: 10 minutes

Servings: *2*

Ingredients:

For Sauce:

- 1 jalapeno pepper
- 1 tablespoon chopped parsley
- 1 teaspoon minced garlic
- 1/2 teaspoon cumin
- 1/2 teaspoon paprika
- 1/2 teaspoon lime zest
- 1 tablespoon honey
- 1 tablespoon lime juice
- 1 tablespoon olive oil
- 1 tablespoon water

For Fish:

- 2 salmon fillets, each about 5 ounces
- 1 cup water
- 1/2 teaspoon salt
- 1/8 teaspoon ground black pepper

Directions:

1. Prepare salmon and for this, season salmon with salt and black pepper until evenly coated.

2. Plugin instant pot, insert the inner pot, pour in water, then place steamer basket and place seasoned salmon on it.

3. Seal instant pot with its lid, press the 'steam' button, then press the 'timer' to set the **Cooking Time**to 5 minutes and cook on high pressure, for 5 minutes.

4. Transfer all the **Ingredients** for the sauce in a bowl, whisk until combined and set aside until required.

5. When the timer beeps, press 'cancel' button and do quick pressure release until pressure nob drops down.

6. Open the instant pot, then transfer salmon to a **Serving** plate and drizzle generously with prepared sauce.

7. Serve straight away.

Nutrition: 305 Calories; 29g Carbohydrates; 6g Fiber

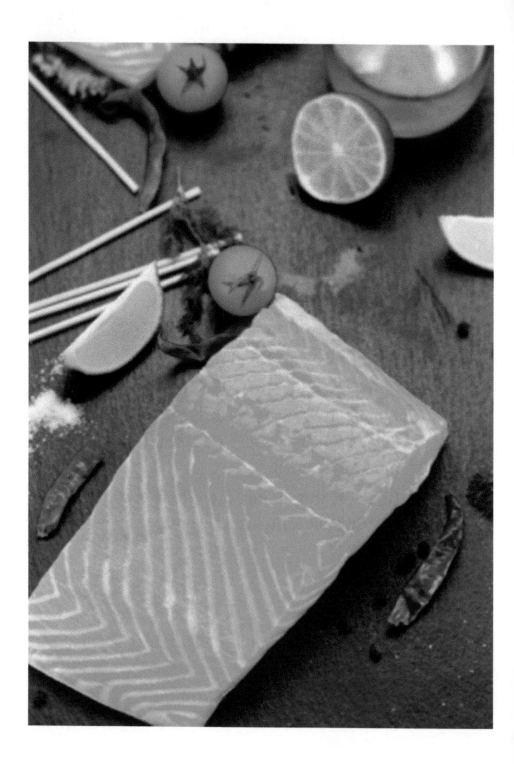

Collard Greens

Preparation Time: 5 minutes

Cooking Time*: 6 hours*

Servings: *12*

Ingredients:

- 2 pounds chopped collard greens
- ¾ cup chopped white onion
- 1 teaspoon onion powder
- 1 teaspoon garlic powder
- 1 teaspoon salt
- 2 teaspoons brown sugar
- ½ teaspoon ground black pepper
- ½ teaspoon red chili powder
- ¼ teaspoon crushed red pepper flakes
- 3 tablespoons apple cider vinegar
- 2 tablespoons olive oil
- 14.5-ounce vegetable broth
- 1/2 cup water

Directions:

1. Plugin instant pot, insert the inner pot, add onion and collard and then pour in vegetable broth and water.

2. Close instant pot with its lid, seal, press the 'slow cook' button, then press the 'timer' to set the **Cooking Time**to 6 hours at high heat setting.

3. When the timer beeps, press 'cancel' button and do natural pressure release until pressure nob drops down.

4. Open the instant pot, add remaining **Ingredients** and stir until mixed.

5. Then press the 'sauté/simmer' button and cook for 3 to minutes or more until collards reach to desired texture.

6. Serve straight away.

Nutrition: 49 Calories; 2.3g Carbohydrates; 0.5g Fiber

Mashed Pumpkin

Preparation Time: 9 minutes

Cooking Time: 15 minutes

Servings: *2*

Ingredients:

- 2 cups chopped pumpkin
- 0.5 cup water
- 2tbsp powdered sugar-free sweetener of choice
- 1tbsp cinnamon

Directions:

1. Place the pumpkin and water in your Instant Pot.
2. Seal and cook on Stew 15 minutes.
3. Remove and mash with the sweetener and cinnamon.

Nutrition: 12 Calories; 3g Carbohydrates; 1g Sugar

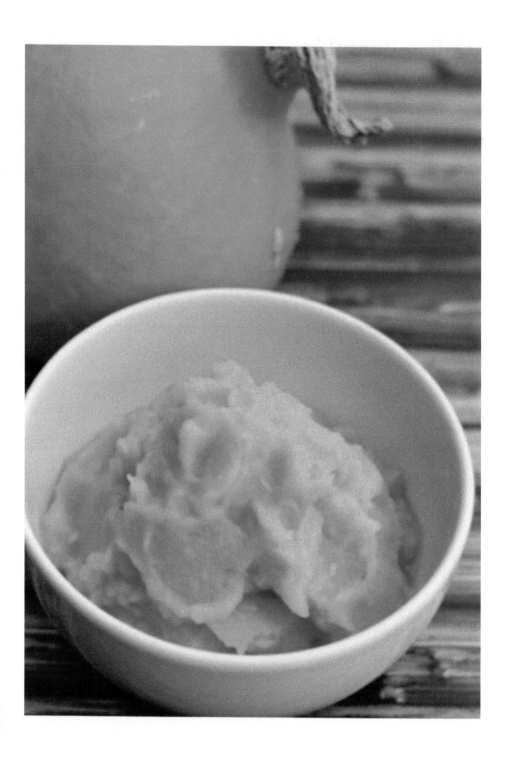

Parmesan-Topped Acorn Squash

Preparation Time: 8 minutes

Cooking Time: 20 minutes

Servings: *4*

Ingredients:

- 1 acorn squash (about 1 pound)
- 1 tablespoon extra-virgin olive oil
- 1 teaspoon dried sage leaves, crumbled
- ¼ teaspoon freshly grated nutmeg
- 1/8 teaspoon kosher salt
- 1/8 teaspoon freshly ground black pepper
- 2 tablespoons freshly grated Parmesan cheese

Directions:

1. Chop acorn squash in half lengthwise and remove the seeds. Cut each half in half for a total of 4 wedges. Snap off the stem if it's easy to do.

2. In a small bowl, combine the olive oil, sage, nutmeg, salt, and pepper. Brush the cut sides of the squash with the olive oil mixture.

3. Fill 1 cup of water into the electric pressure cooker and insert a wire rack or trivet.

4. Place the squash on the trivet in a single layer, skin-side down.

5. Set the lid of the pressure cooker on sealing.

6. Cook on high pressure for 20 minutes.

7. Once done, press Cancel and quick release the pressure.

8. Once the pin drops, open it.

9. Carefully remove the squash from the pot, sprinkle with the Parmesan, and serve.

__Nutrition:__ 85 Calories; 12g Carbohydrates; 2g Fiber

Quinoa Tabbouleh

Preparation Time: 8 minutes

Cooking Time: 16 minutes

Servings: 6

Ingredients:

- 1 cup quinoa, rinsed
- 1 large English cucumber
- 2 scallions, sliced
- 2 cups cherry tomatoes, halved
- 2/3 cup chopped parsley
- 1/2 cup chopped mint
- ½ teaspoon minced garlic
- 1/2 teaspoon salt
- ½ teaspoon ground black pepper
- 2 tablespoon lemon juice
- 1/2 cup olive oil

Directions:

1. Plugin instant pot, insert the inner pot, add quinoa, then pour in water and stir until mixed.

2. Close instant pot with its lid and turn the pressure knob to seal the pot.

3. Select 'manual' button, then set the 'timer' to 1 minute and cook in high pressure, it may take 7 minutes.

4. Once the timer stops, select 'cancel' button and do natural pressure release for 10 minutes and then do quick pressure release until pressure nob drops down.

5. Open the instant pot, fluff quinoa with a fork, then spoon it on a rimmed baking sheet, spread quinoa evenly and let cool.

6. Meanwhile, place lime juice in a small bowl, add garlic and stir until just mixed.

7. Then add salt, black pepper, and olive oil and whisk until combined.

8. Transfer cooled quinoa to a large bowl, add remaining **Ingredients** , then drizzle generously with the prepared lime juice mixture and toss until evenly coated.

9. Taste quinoa to adjust seasoning and then serve.

__Nutrition:__ 283 Calories; 30.6g Carbohydrates; 3.4g Fiber

Wild Rice Salad with Cranberries and Almonds

Preparation Time: 6 minutes

Cooking Time: 25 minutes

Servings: *18*

Ingredients:

For the rice

- 2 cups wild rice blend, rinsed
- 1 teaspoon kosher salt
- 2½ cups Vegetable Broth

For the dressing

- ¼ cup extra-virgin olive oil
- ¼ cup white wine vinegar
- 1½ teaspoons grated orange zest
- Juice of 1 medium orange (about ¼ cup)
- 1 teaspoon honey or pure maple syrup

For the salad

- ¾ cup unsweetened dried cranberries
- ½ cup sliced almonds, toasted
- Freshly ground black pepper

Directions:

1. To make the rice

2. In the electric pressure cooker, combine the rice, salt, and broth.

3. Close and lock the lid. Set the valve to sealing.

4. Cook on high pressure for 25 minutes.

5. When the cooking is complete, hit Cancel and allow the pressure to release naturally for 1minutes, then quick release any remaining pressure.

6. Once the pin drops, unlock and remove the lid.

7. Let the rice cool briefly, then fluff it with a fork.

8. To make the dressing

9. While the rice cooks, make the dressing: In a small jar with a screw-top lid, combine the olive oil, vinegar, zest, juice, and honey. (If you don't have a jar, whisk the **Ingredients** together in a small bowl.) Shake to combine.

10.   To make the salad

11.   Mix rice, cranberries, and almonds.

12.   Add the dressing and season with pepper.

13.   Serve warm or refrigerate.

Nutrition: 126 Calories; 18g Carbohydrates; 2g Fiber

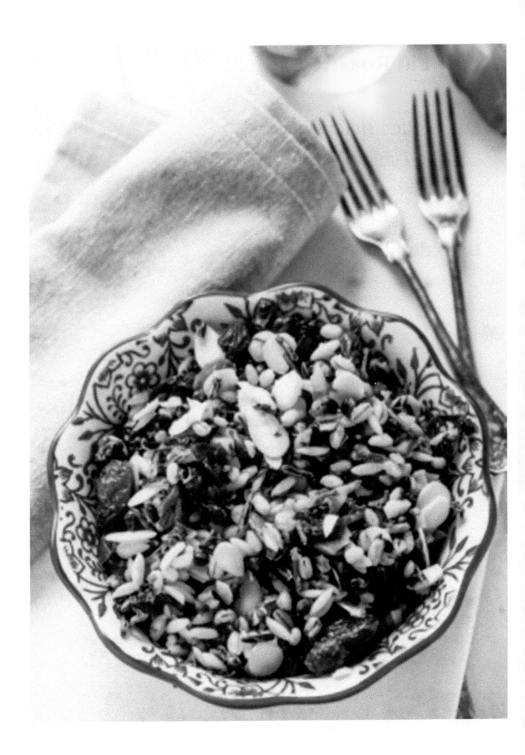

Low Fat Roasties

Preparation Time: 8 minutes

Cooking Time: 25 minutes

Servings: *2*

Ingredients:

- 1lb roasting potatoes
- 1 garlic clove
- 1 cup vegetable stock
- 2tbsp olive oil

Directions:

1. Position potatoes in the steamer basket and add the stock into the Instant Pot.
2. Steam the potatoes in your Instant Pot for 15 minutes.
3. Depressurize and pour away the remaining stock.
4. Set to sauté and add the oil, garlic, and potatoes. Cook until brown.

Nutrition: 201 Calories; 3g Carbohydrates; 6g Fat